CONTENTS

(page numbers)

CHAIRMAN'S FOREWORD

It was a privilege to be invited to chair the first gynaecological meeting organized by the Duphar Medical Relations team and help in the editing of this small book to cover the expert's presentations and lively discussion which followed. This book will provide the reader with a precise account of the epidemiological, aetiological and pathological background knowledge, as well as the role of investigative techniques and the place of surgery, radiotherapy and progesterone therapy in the management of endometrial cancer.

In order to help the reader, all questions which were raised by a member of the audience, or one of the speakers to another, which related to a specific topic have been placed at the end of the appropriate chapter. The more general questions usually answered by more than one expert are brought together in a separate section at the end of the book.

The educational purpose of the meeting will have been beneficial if it makes those attending and all those who read this book reflect in future on each case of endometrial cancer they encounter and follow some of the guidelines mentioned by the experts. I am certain they will all at least be convinced we are too complacent about the present management of endometrial cancer and that we can and must do better.

V R TINDALL
Professor of Obstetrics & Gynaecology
University of Manchester

WP440

Current Approaches

Endometrial Carcinoma

Edited by
J C Malkin & V R Tindall

MEDICAL LIBRARY
WATFORD POSTGRADUATE
MEDICAL CENTRE
WATFORD GENERAL HOSPITAL
VICARAGE ROAD
WATFORD WD1 8HB

**duphar
medical relations**

© 1988 Duphar Laboratories Limited
Gaters Hill, West End,
Southampton SO3 3JD

First published 1988

ISBN 1-870678-04-4

Printed and bound in Great Britain by
Henry Ling Ltd., at the Dorset Press, Dorchester, Dorset

PATHOLOGY OF ENDOMETRIAL CARCINOMA: WITH PARTICULAR REFERENCE TO PROGNOSTIC FACTORS

H Fox
Professor of Reproductive Pathology
University of Manchester

In this contribution the pathological features of endometrial adenocarcinoma that are of prognostic significance will be discussed.

HISTOLOGICAL TYPE

The current classification of endometrial adenocarcinoma is given in Table 1. Basically, the various types of neoplasm that can occur in the endometrium represent the different pathways of differentiation which are open to undifferentiated cells of Müllerian type. Thus differentiation may be along endometrial, endocervical or tubal pathways to give, respectively, endometrioid, mucinous or serous papillary tumours.

TABLE 1
Classification of Carcinoma of Endometrium

1. Endometrioid Adenocarcinoma
   Variants
   a. Papillary
   b. Secretory
   c. Ciliated cell
   d. With squamous differentiation
      (1) Adenocarcinoma with squamous metaplasia (adenoacanthoma)
      (2) Adenosquamous carcinoma
2. Mucinous adenocarcinoma
3. Serous adenocarcinoma
4. Clear cell adenocarcinoma
5. Squamous cell carcinoma
6. Undifferentiated carcinoma
7. Mixed
8. Unclassifiable

The term 'endometrioid adenocarcinoma' describes the usual adenocarcinoma of the endometrium, which accounts for about 85% of all endometrial carcinomas. These tumours often show bland squamous metaplasia, and it is quite common for them to be then classed as 'adenoacanthomas' which are regarded by some as a separate entity having an unusually good prognosis. There is, in fact, no justification for the continued retention of this terminology for it is impossible to define an adenoacanthoma in

1

specific terms (largely because some degree of squamous metaplasia is present in nearly every endometrioid adenocarcinoma) and because it is now known that adenoacanthomas have exactly the same prognosis as do tumours of similar grade which lack squamous metaplasia. It is, however, very important to differentiate bland squamous metaplasia within an endometrioid adenocarcinoma from the malignant squamous epithelium which is seen in an adenosquamous carcinoma. This latter tumour is somewhat controversial, for although some centres in North America have claimed that there has been a considerable increase in the incidence of this neoplasm (up to 30% of all endometrial carcinoma), others have not noted this. Controversy also surrounds its prognosis which is regarded by some as very poor and others as being no different to that of endometrioid adenocarcinoma. Our own experience in Manchester, coincides with that of Christopherson in Kentucky; in neither centre has there been any increase in the incidence of this neoplasm, it remaining stable at about 5 to 6% of all cases of endometrial adenocarcinoma. Further, it was clear from both these series that adenosquamous carcinoma has a poor prognosis and is a relatively lethal form of neoplasia.

Even more lethal is the serous papillary adenocarcinoma which appears to be increasing in frequency and is histologically identical to the serous papillary carcinoma of the ovary. Despite a relatively bland appearance this tumour invades the uterine lymphatics and blood vessels at a very early stage in its evolution, thus resulting in early lymph node metastases. The five year survival rate for women with a serous papillary carcinoma of the endometrium is in the region of only 15%. It is, however, very important to differentiate the true papillary serous adenocarcinoma from the papillary variant of the endometrioid adenocarcinoma, a neoplasm which has a good prognosis.

The clear cell adenocarcinoma of the endometrium is also identical to its ovarian counterpart, and to the clear cell adenocarcinoma of the vagina that occurs in young women exposed antenatally to DES. This tumour also tends to invade lymphatic and vascular spaces at a very early stage in its evolution and is associated with a very poor prognosis.

Mucinous adenocarcinoma of the endometrium is a distinct entity, but difficult to distinguish from endocervical adenocarcinoma unless fractional curettage is carried out. The prognosis for a mucinous adenocarcinoma is exactly the same as is that for the ordinary endometrioid adenocarcinoma.

STAGE

In general terms there is a very good correlation between stage and prognosis for patients with Stage I endometrial adenocarcinoma, which everybody agrees has a good prognosis, and the Stage IV endometrial adenocarcinoma which clearly is associated with a bad prognosis. There is, however, a wide disparity between differing series for the prognosis of patients with Stage II and Stage III neoplasms, this being because of difficulties that are encountered in allotting patients to these particular stages. In allotting a particular neoplasm to Stage II there must be true invasion of the cervical tissues. The mere presence of tumour within the endocervical canal, though often taken to be evidence of cervical involvement, does not mean that a tumour is Stage II; there must be true and definite invasion of the cervical stroma. Even if tumour is spreading along the endocervical cervix this still does not place the tumour at Stage II without concomitant stromal invasion.

In Stage III cases the difficulty arises when there is concomitant ovarian endometrioid adenocarcinoma. Criteria for deciding whether these represent two synchronous primary neoplasms or whether the ovarian tumour is a metastasis from the endometrial neoplasm are not yet fully clarified, so the difficulty is unresolved for many Stage III cases. It is, however, generally true that in most cases these are not true Stage III tumours, but synchronous primary neoplasms.

There are two unfortunate aspects to a slavish adherence to tumour stage as a prognostic feature. Firstly, although most patients with Stage I neoplasms do well and most women with Stage IV neoplasms do badly, it is nevertheless the case that some women with Stage I disease die quite quickly, while others with Stage IV disease remain alive for a long time. Therefore, stage is not a good prognostic indicator for an individual patient. Secondly, although patients with Stage I neoplasms have a good prognosis, the fact is, that because such tumours represent the majority of patients with endometrial adenocarcinoma, most deaths from endometrial adenocarcinoma are in women who present initially with Stage I disease.

It is because of these two latter factors that prognostic features have to be sought which are independent of stage.

GRADE

Tumour grade is recognized to be of prognostic importance. Most pathologists grade endometrial adenocarcinoma in architectural terms, simply as well differentiated, moderately differentiated or poorly differentiated. In Grade I tumours, there is a reasonably good correlation with prognosis, but disagreement arises as to the exact prognosis for patients with Grade II and Grade III neoplasms. There are particular reasons for this in so far as whilst any junior pathologist can recognize a well differentiated or a very poorly differentiated adenocarcinoma, it takes considerable experience to achieve any consistency in distinguishing the borders between, for example, Grade I and Grade II or between Grade II and Grade III. Indeed, these boundaries have never been clearly defined, and tend to be assessed in a highly arbitrary and subjective fashion.

Histological grading in purely architectural terms is insufficiently discriminatory, partly because too many cases fall into the Grade I category and also because no account is taken of cytological atypia. It is of importance, therefore, that the degree of nuclear atypia be taken into account when grading a neoplasm. Thus, if a tumour is Grade I in architectural terms but has a significant degree of nuclear atypia, it should be reallocated to Grade II. This will add a further degree of discrimination to the grading process which still remains, however, highly arbitrary.

DEPTH OF INVASION

In most series there seems to be a reasonably good correlation between prognosis and depth of myometrial invasion. In practise it is far from easy to assess the depth of invasion and, furthermore, we do not really know what we are measuring or why we are measuring it. Is it for instance, the depth from the endomyometrial junction that is important or is it the distance from the serosa which is important? An answer to this question is currently lacking.

LYMPHATIC INVOLVEMENT

We have recently completed a survey of lymphatic involvement and have found it to be an independent prognostic value of great significance. Even in Grade I, Stage I cases which are only superficially invasive, the presence of lymphatic or vascular space involvement implies a poor prognosis and an assessment of this should be an obligatory part of the pathologist's report.

STATE OF NON-NEOPLASTIC ENDOMETRIUM

It is important to note the nature of the non-neoplastic endometrium, for it is now clear that adenocarcinomas arising from a background of 'atypical hyperplasia' have a very much better prognosis than do neoplasms which arise in an atrophic or normal cycling endometrium. The possible implication of this is that we are dealing with two entirely different neoplastic entities, one evolving slowly from a background of 'hyperplasia' and the other arising much more quickly from an atrophic endometrium.

STEROID RECEPTOR STATUS

Steroid receptor status in endometrial carcinomas can now be assessed immunocyto-chemically. The presence or absence of oestrogen receptors in endometrial adenocarcinoma is of some discriminatory value. Tumours with abundant oestrogen receptors have a good prognosis, whereas those with none have a poor prognosis, all the intermediate stages of decreasing density being associated with increasingly poor prognosis.

Progesterone receptor status is highly discriminatory. Those tumours lacking progesterone receptors have a universally poor prognosis whilst those with any density of progesterone receptors tend to have a good prognosis.

TUMOUR MARKERS

A wide range of tumour markers have been studied for their prognostic value in endometrial adenocarcinoma, these including hCG, CEA, CA1, CA125 and various monoclonal antibodies: none of these have proved to be of any prognostic significance. In our own studies of CEA positive reactivity a minor point has emerged, namely, that tumours which are CEA negative tend to respond better to a combination of surgery and radiotherapy than those which are CEA positive. Apart from this subset of cases, however, CEA is of no other prognostic value.

4

FUTURE TRENDS

Morphometry

Pathologists are not able to grade tumours in a meaningful and consistent manner, and it is inevitable, therefore, that machines will be developed that can do so much better. Morphometry is already proving a powerful prognostic tool in many fields of pathology, and it is undoubtedly true that morphometric analysis can detect changes of prognostic significance that escape the light microscopist. As yet, morphometry has not been extensively applied to endometrial adenocarcinoma, but it is reasonably certain that it will eventually prove of considerable discriminatory value, particularly in those cases which are Stage I, Grade I.

Flow Cytometry

Flow cytometry offers a very rapid technique for measuring tumour DNA and hence for measuring the ploidy of the neoplasm. In many tumours elsewhere aneuploidy has been associated with a poor prognosis, certainly worse than that for tumours with normal ploidy. It has not yet been proved that this is necessarily the case for endometrial adenocarcinoma. Flow cytometry can also be used to measure the 'proliferation index', that is, the number of cells which are in the S and G2 phase of the mitotic cycle; preliminary studies indicate a good correlation between this proliferation index and prognosis.

Oncogene Expression

There will undoubtedly be, in the future, many studies of oncogene expression in endometrial adenocarcinoma but they are unlikely to yield results of significant prognostic value.

CONCLUSIONS

The pathological features of an endometrial adenocarcinoma yield many prognostic clues. The histological type, stage, depth of myometrial invasion, the presence of lymphatic space involvement and the nature of the adjacent non-neoplastic endometrium are all of prognostic value. Prognostic indices are further refined by the use of the newer techniques of morphometry and flow cytometry. One of the major problems in gynaecological oncology is the over-emphasis on stage; gynaecologists have become entrapped in this concept, which in fact does not yield prognostic information to the individual patient. Therefore the search must continue for prognostic factors that are independent of, and operate within, a single stage. If all these various factors are taken into account, it does seem to emerge that there are two types of endometrial adenocarcinoma.

1. One commonly arising from a background of hyperplasia, is well differentiated, slowly growing, not deeply invasive, has no great tendency to invade lymphatic or vascular channels and can be treated by the simplest possible measures.

2. The other type of tumour tends to arise from an atrophic endometrium, tends to be poorly differentiated and deeply invasive and is the type of tumour which requires extremely aggressive therapy.

REFERENCE

Christopherson W M (1986). The significance of the pathologic findings in endometrial cancer. *Clinics Obstet. Gynaecol., 13*, 673–693.

FURTHER READING

Beckner M E, Mori T, Silverberg S G (1985). Endometrial carcinoma: nontumor factors in prognosis. *Int. J. Gynecol. Pathol., 4*, 131–145.

Hendrickson M R, Kempson R L (1987). Endometrial hyperplasia, metaplasia and carcinoma. In: Haines and Taylor, Obstetrical and Gynaecological Pathology (ed Fox H), Churchill Livingstone, Edinburgh.

Kadar N R D, Kohorn E I, Livolsi V A, Kapp D S (1982). Histologic variants of cervical involvement by endometrial carcinoma. *Obstet. Gynecol., 59*, 85–92.

Silverberg S G (1984). New aspects of endometrial carcinoma. *Clinics Obstet. Gynaecol., 11*, 189–208.

DISCUSSION—RELATED TO PROFESSOR FOX'S PRESENTATION

Question   Can you use both grading and staging to determine tumour prognosis?

Fox   Yes, by doing a multivariate analysis. However, it is not discriminatory because the majority of Stage I are also Grade I. The multivariate tables show the weighting of each prognostic factor. Grade has much greater weight than stage.

Question   With regard to tumour markers, where are you measuring CEA in the plasma?

Fox   These are not plasma CEA but tumour content of CEA.

Question   What is the natural history of a clear cell carcinoma of the endometrium?

Fox   It behaves as a very rapidly progressive, rapidly spreading and early metastasing virulent adenocarcinoma.

Question   Do cases of clear cell carcinoma occur without metastasing?

Fox   You do come across cases without spread. Even in the Christopherson series of Stage I cases without spread, which were very carefully staged, there is only something like a 40% five year survival rate for the clear cell carcinomas, and they have a very bad prognosis.

ENDOMETRIAL HYPERSTIMULATION WITH EXOGENOUS OESTROGENS

M I Whitehead
Senior Lecturer and Honorary Consultant
Kings College Hospital, London

RISK OF MALIGNANCY

Since the publication of the first papers in 1975 and 1976 reporting an association between exogenous oestrogen use and endometrial carcinoma (Smith et al, 1975; Ziel and Finkle, 1975; Mack et al, 1976) there has been a vast amount of literature on the subject. The association is now known to be both dose-related (Peterson et al, 1986) and dependent on the duration of therapy (Cramer and Knapp, 1979). According to Cramer and Knapp (1979) the cumulative risk of developing endometrial carcinoma in an untreated woman between the ages of 50–65 years is 1% compared with a risk of 7% in a woman treated with unopposed cyclical oestrogen for this 15 year period of time. Expressed slightly differently, 5 women per 1000 women per year exposed to unopposed oestrogen will develop endometrial cancer: the incidence in an untreated population is 1 woman per 1000 women per year.

The effect of exposure to exogenous oestrogens on the subsequent survival appears to be favourable. Comparisons are available for long-term survivors from endometrial cancer by oestrogen use: more previous users survive than non-users (Chu et al, 1982; Elwood and Boyes, 1980). However, comparisons between these groups may not be strictly valid, there being other differences between the users and non-users.

SURGICAL INTERVENTION

Malignancy apart, other aspects of long term unopposed oestrogen therapy deserve consideration. Ettinger et al (in press) showed that 50% of patients on oestrogen therapy over a period of 20 years eventually required curettage compared with 8% of matched controls. The hysterectomy rate was likewise increased with 28% of treated women undergoing hysterectomy for either hyperplasia/carcinoma or irregular bleeding compared with 3% of controls; the latter required surgery mainly due to prolapse. The fact that 1 in 3 women in this study underwent major surgery has considerable cost implications for the planning of health care strategies.

REDUCING THE RISKS OF THERAPY

There are several ways to reduce the incidence of hyperplasia and the development of carcinoma.

Serial biopsy both before and during treatment could be carried out on all patients. However, biopsy causes significant discomfort in the majority of patients (Siddle et al, 1983) and is hardly cost-effective when the maximum pick-up rate is 5 women per 1000 per year of oestrogen exposure. All patients would need to be biopsied since there is no correlation between endometrial status and patterns of vaginal bleeding.

Reduction of the dose of oestrogen has also been proposed, but unless sufficient oestrogen is prescribed hot flushes and other symptoms will not be relieved nor will post-menopausal bone mass be conserved. The oestrogen doses required for symptom relief and conservation of bone mass cause endometrial stimulation. Varying the type of oestrogen has little effect. The theory that oestrone compounds should be avoided due to their carcinogenic properties (Ziel and Finkle, 1976) was discredited when the intranuclear oestrogen in the endometrium of oestrogen-exposed women was shown to be oestradiol (Whitehead *et al*, 1981). The addition of oestriol to oestradiol-based preparations does not reduce the degree of endometrial proliferation (Padwick *et al*, 1986). Continuous oestrogen therapy has no advantages over cyclical oestrogens with regard to preventing the development of hyperplasia (Schiff et al, 1982).

COMBINATION THERAPY

Combination therapy with a progestogen and an oestrogen is currently the most sensible strategy although insufficient epidemiological data has accumulated to date to properly assess the risk of malignancy with this treatment. Early indications, from a prospective study, are that there is no increased risk of hyperplasia on combination therapy (Persson *et al*, 1986) or, from retrospective studies, even a reduced risk of malignancy compared to untreated women and those on unopposed oestrogen therapy (Gambrell, 1986).

Endometrial biopsy, although not cost-effective as a screening procedure, can be valuable in analysing the effects of oestrogens on the endometrium over shorter periods of time. We found that in a group of post-menopausal women on unopposed oestrogen therapy for 18 months, 15–20% developed cystic hyperplasia and a further 5–10% developed atypical hyperplasia. The spontaneous development of endometrial carcinoma from cystic hyperplasia is thought to be approximately 1%, and from atypical hyperplasia about 12–50% depending on the severity of the changes. The addition of progestogens for 7 days in each month reduced the incidence of hyperplasia from an overall 30% to 4% (Whitehead, 1978). When extended to 10 days this was further reduced to 2% and 12 days of progestogens per month abolished hyperplasia completely (Studd *et al*, 1978; Whitehead *et al*, 1982). Clearly the duration of progestogen administration is critical although the optimal treatment duration has yet to be defined. The 7 days per month regimen used in this country may be inadequate—we add progestogens for the first 12 days of each calendar month which is a simple, acceptable routine for most women although some will develop side effects due to the progestogen. These can be symptomatic or psychological and amount to an iatrogenic form of the pre-menstrual syndrome with depression, anxiety, irritability, breast tenderness, bloating or abdominal cramps.

CELLULAR RESPONSES TO COMBINATION THERAPY

Oestrogens increase DNA synthesis within the endometrium and stimulate both oestradiol and progesterone receptor formation. Progestogens have an anti-mitotic effect (suppression of DNA synthesis and receptor formation) and also increase the activity of certain enzymes such as the dehydrogenases. We have examined the effect upon the endometrium of various types and doses of progestogens and we have demonstrated a clear dose-dependent relationship with most. Conjugated equine oestrogens 1.25 mg gave values for DNA synthesis well within the pre-menopausal proliferative phase range. Dydrogesterone in doses of 5, 10 and 20 mg, when added to the conjugated oestrogens and with biopsy on the sixth day of dydrogesterone administration, gave values within the pre-menopausal secretory phase range for the 10 and 20 mg doses. With medroxyprogesterone acetate (MPA) in doses of 2.5, 5 and 10 mg per day, added to conjugated oestrogens 0.625 mg per day, the response was again dose-dependent with the lowest MPA dose giving sub-optimal responses in most patients. It is important to stress that with all progestogens we have observed a wide individual variation in response so it is important, therefore, to examine data as individual observations rather than as means and standard errors. Histologically there was also a wide range of responses with some patients achieving wholly secretory endometrium with the lowest progestogen doses but with others having partially secretory or even proliferative features. What we needed, therefore, was a simple non-invasive test to determine how well each individual patient was responding to the progestogen that we prescribed.

As the dose of progestogen is reduced, we noticed that some patients began to bleed earlier each month. We investigated this further by asking 102 women on combination therapy to record the day of onset of vaginal bleeding for 3 months, thus giving a mean, then performing an endometrial biopsy on the sixth day of therapy in the fourth month. The 17 women with proliferative endometria had all bled by day 10 of progestogen addition (day 1 was the first day of added progestogen) whereas the 54 women with secretory endometria had all bled on day 11 or later. In the group with mixed patterns, those in whom proliferative endometrium predominated had bled early and vice versa. A small group were unsuitable for assessment. This pattern has been found with each oestrogen and progestogen that we have examined. Those who reported bleeding by day 9 or 10 have proliferative endometrium and those who bleed after day 12 are in the secretory phase (Padwick *et al*, 1986).

METABOLIC EFFECTS OF COMBINATION THERAPY

One of the major criticisms of progestogen use is their potentially adverse metabolic effects. Progesterone itself influences carbohydrate metabolism: most of its derivatives behave likewise and some also affect lipid and lipoprotein metabolism. Evidence is now accumulating showing that it is impossible to reduce the potentially adverse metabolic effects of progestogens by reducing the dose.

Some workers, but not all (Padwick *et al*, 1986), believe that progestogens may influence the risk of arterial disease by altering the proportions of HDL and LDL cholesterol in plasma: increased HDL and decreased LDL are currently believed to be beneficial. HDL increases in a dose-related manner as the dose of post-menopausal oestrogen is increased (Jensen *et al*, 1986) and the addition of norethisterone 1 mg per day, for 10 days, whilst reducing the HDL level overall by 4–6%, did not suppress it below baseline (pre-treatment) levels. Higher doses of norethisterone, 10 mg per day, cause significant suppression of HDL cholesterol (Hirvonen *et al*, 1981). It may thus be possible to provide endometrial safety with minimal adverse metabolic effects.

CONTINUOUS COMBINED THERAPY

Whilst symptomatic women will tolerate the re-establishment of regular withdrawal bleeding, it has been argued that those who are asymptomatic and on HRT for preservation of bone mass are less tolerant. By adding a progestogen every day it should, theoretically, be possible to avoid bleeding by converting the proliferative endometrium into atrophic endometrium. Staland (1981) and Mattsson and colleagues (1982) both reported continuing problems with chronic light bleeding or spotting in up to 40% of their group of patients over the first 6 months. Magos *et al* (1985) increased the progestogen dose if bleeding occurred, eventually achieving amenorrhoea over a 12–15 month period in all remaining patients but drop-out rates were high, 50% of those taking 1.25 mg of conjugated equine oestrogens daily and 25% of those on the 0.625 mg per day dose. Our own prospective, randomised study over 6 months using twice daily progestogen has had a 20% drop out rate (Whitehead, 1986). Some women do well on continuous combined therapies and achieve amenorrhoea soon after treatment commences; in others chronic light bleeding persists and eventually deters them and there is no way of predicting the response. Neither do we have any information yet on the relationship between continuous combined therapy and the development of malignancy.

REFERENCES

Chu J, Schweid A I, Weiss N S (1982). Survival among women with endometrial cancer: a comparison of estrogen users and non-users. *Am. J. Obstet. Gynecol.*, *143*, 569.

Cramer D W, Knapp R C (1979). Review of epidemiologic studies of endometrial cancer and exogenous oestrogen. *Obstet. Gynecol.*, *54*, 521.

Elwood J M, Boyes D A (1980). Clinical and pathological features and survival of endometrial cancer patients in relation to prior use of estrogens. *Gynaecol. Oncol.*, *10*, 173.

Ettinger B, Golditch I M, Friedman G (In Press). Gynecologic consequences of long-term estrogen replacement therapy.

Gambrell R D Jr (1986). Prevention of endometrial cancer with progestogens. *Maturitas*, *8*, 159.

Hirvonen E, Malkonen M, Manninen·V (1981). Effects of different progestogens on lipoproteins during postmenopausal replacement therapy. *New Engl. J. Med.*, *304*, 560–563.

Jensen J, Nilas L, Christiensen C (1986). Cyclic changes in serum cholesterol and lipoproteins following different doses of combined postmenopausal hormone replacement therapy. *Br. J. Obstet. Gynaecol.*, *93*, 613.

Mack T, Pike M, Henderson B, Pfeffer R, Gerkins V, Arthur M, Brown W (1976). Oestrogens and endometrial cancer in a retirement community. *New Engl. J. Med.*, *294*, 1262–1267.

Magos A L, Brincat M, Studd J W W *et al* (1985). Amenorrhoea and endometrial atrophy with continuous oral estrogen and progestogen therapy in postmenopausal women. *Obstet. Gynaecol.*, *65*, 496.

Mattsson L-A, Cullberg G, Samsioe G (1982). Evaluation of a continuous oestrogen-progestogen regimen for climacteric complaints. *Maturitas*, *4*, 95.

Padwick M L, Pryse-Davies J, Whitehead M I (1986). A simple method for determining the optimal dosage of progestin in postmenopausal women receiving estrogens. *New Engl. J. Med.*, *315*, 930–934.

Padwick M L, Siddle N C, Lane G et al (1986). Oestriol with oestradiol versus oestradiol alone: a comparison of endometrial, symptomatic and psychological effects. Br. J. Obstet. Gynaecol., 93, 606.

Persson I R, Adami H-O, Eklund G, Johansson E D B, Lindberg B S, Lindgren A (1986). The risk of endometrial neoplasia and treatment with estrogens and estrogen-progestogen combinations. Acta Obstet. Gynecol. Scand., 65, 211–217.

Peterson H B, Lee N C, Rubin G L (1986). Genital neoplasia. In Mishell D R Jr (ed): Menopause: Physiology and Pharmacology. Chicago, Year Book Medical Publishers Inc.

Schiff I, Sela H K, Cramer D et al (1982). Endometrial hyperplasia in women on cyclic or continuous estrogen regimens. Fertil. Steril., 37, 79.

Siddle N C, Young O, Sledmere C M et al (1983). A controlled trial of naproxen sodium for relief of pain associated with Vabra suction curettage. Br. J. Obstet. Gynaecol., 90, 864.

Smith D C, Prentice R, Thompson D, Herrman W (1975). Association of exogenous oestrogens and endometrial carcinoma. New Engl. J. Med., 293, 1164–1167.

Staland B (1981). Continuous treatment with natural oestrogens and progestogens. A method to avoid endometrial stimulation. Maturitas, 3, 145.

Studd J W W, Thom M H, Paterson M E L et al (1978). The prevention and treatment of endometrial pathology in postmenopausal women receiving exogenous oestrogens. In Pasetto N, Paoletti R, Ambrus J L (eds): The Menopause and Postmenopause. Lancaster, England, MTP Press Ltd.

Whitehead M I (1978). The effects of oestrogens and progestogens on the postmenopausal endometrium. Maturitas, 1, 87.

Whitehead M I (1986). Prevention of endometrial abnormalities. In: Greenblatt R B (ed): A Modern Approach to the Perimenopausal Years. Berlin, de Gruyter.

Whitehead M I, Lane G, Dyer G et al (1981). Oestradiol: the predominant intranuclear oestrogen in the endometrium of oestrogen-treated postmenopausal women. Br. J. Obstet. Gynaecol., 88, 914.

Whitehead M I, Townsend P T, Pryse-Davies J et al (1982). Effects of various types and dosages of progestogens on the postmenopausal endometrium. J. Reprod. Med., 27, 539.

Ziel H, Finkle W (1975). Increased risk of endometrial carcinoma among users of conjugated oestrogens. New Engl. J. Med., 293, 1167–1170.

Ziel H K, Finkle W D (1976). Association of estrone and the development of endometrial cancer. Am. J. Obstet. Gynecol., 124, 735.

DISCUSSION—RELATED TO MR WHITEHEAD'S PRESENTATION

Question   Is there any point in adding progestogen to HRT in a patient who has had a hysterectomy for a non-malignant condition?

Whitehead   Gambrell's study shows that in patients taking combination therapy the observed incidence of breast cancer is reduced but there are major methodological flaws in this study and the data cannot justify that conclusion. Tom Anderson's data shows that in the secretory phase, breast epithelial DNA synthesis is suppressed. At present, we do not have any good epidemiological data showing progestogen addition protects against breast cancer and that is the only reason for giving progestogens to a hysterectomised patient. Also there is no good biochemical data showing that progestogens do in breast tissue what they do in endometrial tissue. We do not routinely add progestogens to oestrogen therapy in hysterectomised women.

Question   In a patient who developed Stage I Grade I endometrial carcinoma following oestrogen therapy, would you give her oestrogen again after treatment?

Whitehead   Yes, the smallest dose possible with progestogen cover as well.

Question   A Manchester GP pill survey showed a massive increase in CVA's for women over the age of 35, which was particularly related to norethisterone. Has there been any more data on that?

Whitehead   It is quite invalid to extrapolate pill data to the HRT situation because synthetic oestrogens do cause much more marked effects on fibrinolytic and coagulation mechanisms compared with natural oestrogens. Synthetic oestrogens are not rapidly detoxified by intracellular mechanisms. The HRT data of the 10 or so studies published in the literature report no increase in incidence of venous thromboembolic disease. We do not know what oestrogen/progestogen combination therapy in postmenopausal women is satisfactory. We need to find the progestogen which will be endometrial protective and will minimise metabolic effects.

Question   Which progestogen is the best?

Whitehead   It is all related to dose. Duphaston 10–20 mg daily gives good secretory endometrium but we need nice lipid data which are not yet available. It is not true to say that MPA is devoid of metabolic effects. Otterson's group in Sweden showed that low dose norethisterone gives good endometrial protection in most patients and seems to be associated with minimal effects. We need to look at substances such as oral progesterone and progestogens given by other routes, because if you give a non-oral progestogen you may avoid hepatic metabolism and obviate unwanted metabolic side effects.

Question   Would you ignore the finding on curettage of normal secretory endometrium in a menopausal woman?

Whitehead   I would not be so concerned if it was secretory endometrium because that indicates the presence of endogenous progesterone.

ENVIRONMENTAL CAUSES, ENDOCRINE AND OTHERWISE IN THE CAUSATION OF ENDOMETRIAL CANCER

A P Bond

Consultant Gynaecologist

Princess Margaret Hospital, Swindon

The archetypal image of the patient with endometrial cancer is a women in her 50's or 60's, obese and nulliparous with a complicated menstrual history culminating in a late menopause. She is also likely to have uterine fibroids and an impaired glucose tolerance curve. Yet how common is she?

EXTERNAL ENVIRONMENTAL FACTORS

Incidence

All malignancies have increased in incidence this century and disease patterns have changed. In 1900 the ratio of carcinoma of the uterine body to carcinoma of the cervix was 1:8 and by 1970 it was 1:1. Increased life expectancy, family spacing, family size and diagnostic precision have probably all contributed to these changes but cannot account for the increasing incidence since 1970.

Epidemiological analysis shows a suburban preponderance of the disease, equally distributed across all socio-economic groups. Populations vary widely in their incidence with the lowest average found in Japan (1.3 per 100 000) and the highest incidence in the United States (35 per 100 000). Racial factors are important, the incidence in white women being twice that found in black women. Marital status is also significant. The peak incidence occurs in the age group 50 to 70 with some evidence for decreased risk in the over 80's. Menopausal status is less important with the last menstrual period being a relatively insignificant endocrine event in the spectrum of the climacteric.

Diet

The high fat diet of the Western world has been implicated as a factor in the higher incidence of malignancy in these communities (Armstrong and Doll, 1975) and in Japan, where an increasingly sophisticated life-style has not been accompanied by an increased incidence of disease; the diet remains traditionally fish based. However, when Japanese communities move to Western domiciles they soon acquire the higher disease incidences seen there.

Genetics

Endometrial carcinoma was once believed to be inherited as a Mendelian dominant. However, the current thinking is that certain individuals inherit the *tendency* to malignancy, or obesity or other endocrinopathies.

Viruses

Although viral transmission is not implicated in endometrial carcinoma the archetypal woman may be predisposed to viral infection. Endometrial carcinoma has been stimulated to grow in mice using inactivated herpes simplex 1 and 2 virus (Wentz *et al*, 1981).

INTERNAL ENVIRONMENTAL FACTORS

Endocrinopathy

Impaired glucose tolerance frequently accompanies endometrial carcinoma but cancer of all types is more common in diabetics, particularly in insulin-dependent diabetics. When carefully matched, no differences in family history of diabetes or glucose tolerance are detectable between endometrial cancer sufferers and controls. Obesity is more common, the always obese being at higher risk than the recently obese. Again many cancers increase with obesity but few have a particularly convincing endocrine background to them. It may well be that obesity represents a separate risk factor of a non-endocrine variety. Fertility is very difficult to assess retrospectively but in that small sub-set of women who wanted to conceive but remained nulliparous there is certainly a raised incidence of disease compared with controls. Hypertension has never been convincingly separated from obesity in studies of endometrial cancer. Overall, significant differences only exist in obesity and fertility and obesity may well be an independent risk factor.

Sex Steroids

Sex steroid hormones are present in the body from 8–10th week of fetal life and it is difficult to imagine they can become carcinogenic. Although superficially similar to the carcinogens dibenzanthracene and benzpyrene, the steroid molecule lacks the inner aromatic ring associated with carcinogenicity. It is much more likely that oestrogen influences the neoplastic process in some way once it has been initiated by another process and there are several hypotheses about how the initial stem cell mutation arises. Others would argue (Gambrell, 1979) that it is not an excess of oestrogen but a chronic lack of progesterone which is significant.

The Evidence for Oestrogenic Bias

Hypothalamo—Pituitary Axis
There is no convincing evidence at the moment for any difference in the signals between sufferers and controls although new information on pulsatility may well be worth further assessment.

Gonadal and Adrenal Hormone Production
There is quite a lot of evidence to weigh up here:-
    the circumstantial evidence for over-production of oestrogens

the evidence that oestrogen secreting tumours can cause hyperplasia and sometimes eventually adenocarcinoma

endometrial cancer arising from the chronic anovulatory state of the polycystic ovarian syndrome

the effects of relative progesterone deficiency on vaginal smears which often appear oestrogenic in these circumstances

the protective effect of oral contraceptives taken in earlier life

Cortico-stromal hyperplasia of both the ovary and the adrenal has been noted in association with endometrial carcinoma but these are such common phenomena in all post-mortem specimens that no serious conclusions can be drawn. Raised 4-androstenedione, an important precursor for oestradiol, oestrone and testosterone has been found in endometrial cancer sufferers, but when body mass is allowed for in these poorly controlled studies the differences are reduced and often disappear altogether. In my own studies, I could find no detectable differences in glandular production of progesterone, and plasma levels at the time of diagnosis were identical in sufferers and controls.

Peripheral Conversion

This has been thought to occur solely in fat tissue which has propagated the epidemio-logical link with obesity. Certainly fat can convert androstenedione to oestrone and oestrone to oestradiol but more recent work (Jasonni *et al*, 1981) suggests that this does not happen as much as was postulated in obese people. Most of the conversion may actually occur in the liver which is not particularly different in sufferers and controls. However, these three aspects—increased conversion of androstenedione to oestrone, raised oestrone, and possibly decreased oestriol may all exert an oestrogenic effect. When examined critically all of these studies lack controls for at least one of the important epidemiological parameters and when these are corrected for they tend to show minimal or no differences between sufferers and controls.

Plasma Transport Phase

This is a particularly interesting aspect of the hormone signal delivery process because of the great potential for manipulation and amplification of the signal which has already been generated. How a steroid signal is delivered to target tissues is still a matter for debate.

The plasma steroid hormones circulate in three states. A proportion are bound to specific sex hormone binding globulins (e.g. SHBG), another fraction is loosely bound to albumin and some remains unbound. It is this unbound fraction which is believed by most to represent the hormone available for target tissue uptake and metabolism.

Research into the plasma transport phase is a relatively new area and has not as yet yielded much by way of hard data for increased oestrogenicity in those with endo-metrial carcinoma. SHBG and plasma free oestradiol have been found to be lower in cancer sufferers (Davidson *et al*, 1981) but again, once differences in body mass were corrected for the observed differences between patients and controls disappeared. I, too, have found decreased SHBG levels in cancer patients which implies that there is more free fraction available for dissociation diffusion into the cell. However, this was not substantiated by the calculations of free steroids in the same women. Furthermore,

15

such a difference should have persisted along the whole chain of the signal but it did not. I therefore concluded that this was a type 1 statistical error.

Endometrial Uptake

Various possibilities exist. The signal being delivered may be quite ordinary but it may be the endometrium itself which interprets the message in a way that is oestrogenic. It is important when looking at target tissue uptake to assess both the steroid molecule-receptor complex and the enzymic activity within the cell together and this is not easy.

Most researchers in this area have been trying to correlate receptor status with grade of tumour. There have been no really convincing comparisons between normal endo-metrial variants and malignant endometrial grades. The evidence we have shows a slight bias towards oestrogenic behaviour of these cells. In terms of intracellular metabolism, there is some evidence that 17-beta-hydroxysteroid conversion within the cell is different in the endometrium of cancer sufferers compared with normal endometrium. The main conclusion at this stage is that there is no direct evidence of inappropriate oestrogenic activity within the malignant endometrial cell.

CONCLUSION

Apart from the special group of hypo-oestrogenic patients treated for long periods with unopposed exogenous oestrogens, any measurable oestrogenic tendencies in the cancer-prone woman relate more to obesity than to the disease itself. A study of environmental influences thus advances our understanding of the condition and offers the potential for identifying markers of either pre-malignant or early invasive disease. A risk group can be identified from such a study but the endocrine story remains obscure.

REFERENCES

Armstrong B K, Doll R (1975). Environmental factors and cancer incidence and mortality in different countries with special reference to dietary practices. *Int. J. Cancer, 15*, 617–631.
Davidson B J, Gambore J C, Lagane L D, Castaldo T W, Hammond G L, Suteri P K, Judd H L (1981). Free estradiol in post-menopausal women with and without endometrial cancer. *J. Clin. Endocrinol. Metab., 52*, 404–408.
Gambrell R D (1979). The role of hormones in the etiology of breast and endometrial cancer. *Acta Obstet. Gynaecol. Scand., 88*, 73–81.
Jasonni V M, Lodi S, Preti S, Bulletti C, Bonavia M, Bolelli A, Francheschetti F, Flamigni C (1981). Extraglandular oestrogen production in post-menopausal women with and without endometrial cancer: comparison between in vivo and in vitro results. *Cancer Det. Prev. 4*, 469–475.
Wentz W B, Reagan J W, Heggie A D, Fu Y, Anthony D D (1981). Induction of uterine cancer with inactivated herpes simplex virus types 1 and 2. *Cancer, 48*, 1783–1790.

DISCUSSION—RELATED TO MR BOND'S PRESENTATION

Question   What should be the management of women at risk?

Bond   Regular evaluation is mandatory and would enable you to be conservative but at the same time vigilant.

16

MAGNETIC RESONANCE IMAGING

E M Symonds

Professor of Obstetrics and Gynaecology

University Hospital, Queen's Medical Centre, Nottingham

Magnetic resonance imaging has considerable potential in the management of carcinoma of the body of the uterus. The application of a new sophisticated imaging technique to the pre-operative staging of a neoplasm is without value if it can have no effect on the therapeutic decisions.

Patients chosen for examination should fulfil the following criteria:

1. The patient should be at risk of undergoing clinically occult disease that is not obviously apparent on clinical examination.
2. The method should be highly sensitive to the mode of spread at issue.
3. Successful detection of such spread will necessitate different therapeutic measures than would be applied if no spread were encountered.

Clinical examination forms the basis for the staging of endometrial cancer as determined by FIGO in 1982. The stage is based on findings obtained by inspection and palpation including examination under anaesthesia and also the information obtained from fractional curettage, cystoscopy or proctoscopy and the results of radiological studies of the chest, skeleton and urinary tract. Clinical examination may well be normal in the early stages of the disease, as the uterine size and configuration may be quite unchanged. Clinical assessment of direct spread may be hindered by obesity and uterine enlargement caused by fibroids.

Current radiological techniques for the assessment of patients with endometrial carcinoma are of limited value but whilst they are employed to assist in the staging of tumour they rarely contribute to its detection. The yield of tumour-related abnormalities that can be detected by an intravenous ureterogram, chest X-ray and skeletal X-rays is low. There has been little literature with regard to the incidence of IVU abnormalities in association with endometrial cancer. Klempner (1952) quote high rates of hydronephrosis in association with endometrial cancer, but their figures cannot be regarded as representative because their series was small and selective.

A chest X-ray is a necessary base-line investigation, though the incidence of pulmonary metastases is rare. However, with disseminated disease they do occur in 35% to 37% of patients. Both angiography and hysterography were popular in the past, but the results have generally been disappointing and these investigations have now been abandoned. Lymphangiography has been used in several series of patients treated with radiation therapy alone. Although histological proof was rarely obtained it was demonstrated that patients with positive lymphangiograms had a survival rate considerably worse than patients with negative lymphangiograms.

Computer tomography depicts endometrial cancer either as a hypo-dense lesion in the uterine parenchyma, as a fluid-filled uterus due to tumour obstruction in the endo-cervical cavity or vagina, or as a contrast enhancing centre in a hypo-dense lesion.

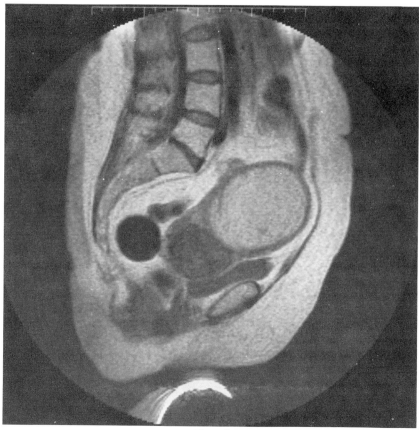

Figure 1
A 54 year old lady with an invasive endometrial adenocarcinoma (high signal area). Inferior to which is a benign leiomyoma (low signal area).

These findings, however, are non-specific and easily confused with leiomyomata, intra-uterine fluid collection and extension of cervical carcinoma into the uterine body. Engelshoven (1983) concluded that the only reliable finding with CT scanning was if a lucency was demonstrated that was more than 35% of the uterine diameter. He concluded CT to be of limited value in Stage I and Stage II disease where clinical assessment was slightly better, but it was considered superior to clinical staging in detecting metastatic carcinoma to omentum and lymph nodes and in the detection of recurrent disease.

Ultrasound is insufficiently accurate in detecting malignant from benign causes of uterine enlargement. There appear to be no diagnostic criteria for endometrial cancer, but there are statistically significant differences in uterine shape and echo pattern between Stage I and II and Stage III and IV disease. False positive diagnoses are caused by leiomyomata creating lobular uterine shape.

18

Magnetic resonance imaging is a new technique which employs the use of radio-frequency radiation in a carefully structured magnetic field. Images can be created in all planes which essentially represent distribution density maps of protons and their related parameters as the so-called T_1 and T_2 relaxation times that are measured in this technique in water and lipids.

By varying the pattern of radiofrequency applied in the so-called pulse sequences, it is possible to weight the images to reflect proton density or T_1 or T_2 elements of the tissues. Magnetic resonance imaging is thereby able to offer a potential for tissue characterisation not associated with other imaging techniques. In addition it employs non-ionising radiofrequency radiation and when used appropriately is without known biological hazard. A T_2 weighted image of the uterus shows that the endometrium has a high signal intensity as distinct from the myometrium which is split into a low intensity inner band and an outer intensity intermediate zone. The low intensity band runs around the endometrial cavity and into the cervix. The nature of this band is unknown but is believed to represent a compacted layer of muscle on the inner aspect of the myometrium. This is of importance in relation to the assessment of endometrial cancers.

Findings

In Nottingham we have used magnetic resonance to examine 46 patients with recurrent and primary endometrial cancer. Endometrial cancer has with a T_2 weighted sequence a high signal intensity similar to that of normal endometrium, but shows some variability. This depends on whether the tumour is diffuse or polypoid and if the endometrial cavity has been distended with a haematometra, or pyometra. Smaller tumours in post-menopausal women have a homogeneous high signal intensity which distinguishes them from the surrounding myometrium. A much larger tumour may have a more intermediate signal intensity.

If a T_1 weighted sequence is now employed the tumour tissue is not highlighted in the same way, but it is now possible to differentiate the tumour from the fluid within the uterine cavity. In the pre-menopausal woman it may be impossible to differentiate tumour from adenomatous hyperplasia or normal endometrium.

Demonstration of an intact low intensity band is, therefore, important in the magnetic resonance assessment of tumour invasion into the myometrium. In three patients the tumour was assessed by magnetic resonance imaging to be confined to the uterine cavity as determined by an intact low intensity band. This assessment was shown to be correct in the hysterectomy specimen in two cases, but in one case there was microscopic superficial invasion. The low intensity band is a fascinating structure, as in a control group of post-menopausal women that we have examined, the band was not visible after the age of 60 years, whereas in the patients with endometrial cancer, the band was observed in 33% of the patients examined whose mean age was 64. The presence of the band is closely related to the oestrogen status of the patient and its presence in the post-menopausal group of women may reflect the hormonal environment of the patient providing an albeit tenuous link between oestrogen and endometrial cancer.

A surgical Stage II tumour had only microscopic tumour invasion of the cervix which was not apparent with MRI nor was visible on gross inspection by the pathologist. In the two cases of Stage III disease, MRI demonstrated tumour tissue to have breached the serosa of the uterus. In three of the four cases of Stage IV, extensive extra-uterine deposits were seen. In two cases of Stage IV tumour omental deposits were demonstrated by the pathologist which was not apparent on the MRI. An excellent correlation was found between the macroscopic pathological assessment of invasion and that demonstrated by the MRI.

As only one patient in our study group underwent a pelvic lymphadenectomy, it has not been possible to address the potential of MRI to detect lymphatic involvement. The potential for magnetic resonance imaging to detect lymphatic involvement because of the high signal intensity associated with a metastasis is certainly feasible.

CONCLUSION

The magnetic resonance imaging provides a unique method of pre-operative assessment of patients with endometrial cancer. Its value may be to assist in directing those cases which require pelvic and para-aortic node biopsy and may allow a re-evaluation of the role of pre-operative radiotherapy. The characteristic signal associated with recurrent tumour may allow its earlier recognition, with the possibility of more effective treatment.

REFERENCES

Engelshoven J M S (1983). Cervical cancer in computed tomography in gynaecological malignancies, Uitgeverij Publifan Maastricht.
Klempner E (1952). Gynaecological lesions and ureterohydronephrosis. *Am. J. Obstet. Gynecol.* *64*, pp. 1232–1241.

DISCUSSION—RELATED TO PROFESSOR SYMOND'S PRESENTATION

Question   Would you routinely carry out MRI on every suspected endometrial cancer patient, and if so why?

Symonds   Yes. We have seen sufficient number of cases where the depth of invasion or the nature of the tumour is sufficiently unexpected on our clinical evaluation to make it useful in pre-operative planning. Whether that is as yet useful in determining outcome of therapy is another issue.

Question   How did that affect your pre-operative planning and what did you do as a result of the findings?

Symonds   The depth of tumour invasion rather than the degree of tumour spread, in some instances, influenced the question of pre-operative radiotherapy as opposed to progestogen therapy, or whether we simply went ahead and did a straightforward hysterectomy.

Question Have you sufficient confidence now to stop doing curettage on women with post-menopausal bleeding, unless the picture suggests a carcinoma?

Symonds No, simply because here I am presenting those cases with proven carcinomas. I could not say that the number of women scanned with post-menopausal bleeding would enable us to say at this point in time that we could reliably replace curettage with scan.

Question Do you envisage that MRI may be used as a screening technique in the future?

Symonds Possibly.

Question Do you use MRI technique to measure endometrial thickness and at what endometrial thickness do you diagnose endometrial carcinoma in a post-menopausal lady?

Symonds Yes we use MRI to measure endometrial thickness and we have done studies on menstrual cycles to establish normal thickness ranges. We would not use thickness measurement as the basis for deciding whether a patient had a carcinoma or whether it was invasive. We also study invasion through the non-resonant band on the inner part of the sub-endometrial zone. In pre-menopausal women it can be very difficult to differentiate between adenomatous hyperplasia, a non-invasive lesion or an early carcinoma.

Question What would you expect the endometrium to be in the post-menopausal woman?

Symonds In the normal post-menopausal women you see a uniform density in the uterus with no band of reduced intensity and an extremely thin endometrial layer. Any thickening would be suspicious of either hyperplastic endometrium or carcinoma.

Question What degree of thickness?

Symonds Anything greater than 2 or 3 millimeters thick would be suspicious.

HYSTEROSCOPY IN ENDOMETRIAL CARCINOMA

Kankipati Shanti Raju

Senior Lecturer and Honorary Consultant

St Thomas' Hospital Medical School, London

The increasing evidence of endometrial carcinoma during the past two decades has restimulated gynaecologists to diagnose this tumour in its early stages, Silverberg (1980), Welch and Scully (1977). Hofmeister (1974) reviewed 20 677 endometrial biopsies and found 187 endometrial carcinomas. Thirty-two of the cases (17%) were totally asymptomatic. This number of unsuspected tumours is indeed significant and warrants a reliable technique for both diagnosis and screening of women at high risk for endometrial carcinoma.

Hysteroscopy is the direct visualisation of the uterine cavity using a fibreoptic endoscope and a cold light source. The first hysteroscopic examination in a live patient was performed as early as 1869 by Pantaleoni. Since then various modifications of the technique of hysteroscopy and its uses have been reported. Its popularity has been waxing and waning for over a century.

The role of hysteroscopy in the management of endometrial carcinoma can be catagorised into:

—Diagnosis
—Staging
—Assessment of tumour size and site
—Direct biopsy
—Screening

Diagnosis

Accuracy is a fundamental feature of any diagnostic test. Although many authorities maintain that dilatation and curettage (D & C) or fractional curettage are by far the most reliable technique, this assertion appears to be lacking.

The sensitivity and specificity of D & C are difficult to assess unless the results of pathologic examination of surgically removed uteri immediately after the D & C, are available. Only one study, by Stock and Kanbour (1975) evaluated the completeness with which samples of endometrium were obtained in D & C's performed immediately before hysterectomy. In their study 30 of 50 patients (60%) had less than half the uterine cavity curetted. This points out the potentially dangerous problem of missing the tumour in the uterine cavity with conventional D & C. Even an experienced gynaecologist curettes at the best 70 to 80% of the endometrium. Direct visualisation of the uterine cavity with a hysteroscope minimises the risk of missing a small, localised area of tumour and facilitates direct biopsy of the tumour for histological confirmation.

TABLE 1
Comparison of Clinical and Surgical Staging in Patients with Endometrial Carcinoma
(Fractional Curettage)

Author	No. of Patients	False Positive	True Positive	False Negative
Wallin *et al* (1984) (Mayo Clinic)	46	39% (18)	61% (28)	
Cowles *et al* (1985) (Kansas Medical Center)	62	50% (31)		13% (6)
Calkins *et al.* (1986) (Indiana University)	81	68.2%		6% (5)

Staging

The reliable clinical staging of endometrial carcinoma remains an unresolved problem. Accurate staging of any malignant condition is important in both planning treatment and evaluating results. Several clinical methods for staging of endometrial carcinoma are currently used. As the majority of women with endometrial carcinoma seek medical attention in early stages, it is crucial to identify Stage I from Stage II as prognosis for Stage II endometrial carcinoma at present is far worse than for Stage I. One of the problems is assessment of endocervical involvement. Fractional curettage is still used by many gynaecologists as a staging procedure. Table 1 shows three recent studies reported from different centres in the United States showing the fallacy of fractional curettage. Clinical staging can be sharpened by assessment of tumour spread at the time of diagnosis by routinely using the hysteroscope. Pre-operative evaluation of the tumour spread at the time of diagnosis has frequently been shown to underestimate extent of the disease (Chen, 1985). Although conventional Stage II requires stromal and glandular involvement of the cervix as important criteria, there is now evidence to show that occult cervical involvement has a 5 year survival similar to Stage I, but it is the gross cervical extension which has a worse prognosis as shown in Table 2. This important clinical prognostic factor can be ascertained at the time of diagnosis by direct viewing of the endocervix with the hysteroscope.

Assessment of size and site of tumour

Both tumour volume and site have a significant effect on prognosis. In 1978 Trotnow *et al* presented their results which showed the 5 year survival for patients with a tumour size of <1 cm was 91.9% for <1.5 cm 88.5% but only 20.6% in patients with tumour larger than 1.5 cm. The preliminary results from staging protocol of the gynaecology oncology group indicate that when isthmus/cervix or both poles of the uterus are involved, there is a rise in the extrauterine spread from 19.1% to 46.2% (Lewis and Bundy, 1981). Hysteroscopy at the time of diagnosis will allow the assessment of both tumour site and size and influence the planning of definitive treatment.

TABLE 2
Stage II Endometrial Carcinoma (Prognosis)

Author	Type of Cervical Spread	No. of Patients	5 year Survival (%)
Surwit et al (1979) (Duke University NC)	No invasion of cervical stroma	39	74
	Invasion of cervical stroma	78	47
Homesley et al (1977) (Memorial Sloan-Kettering NY)	Occult	66	89
	Gross	24	57

TABLE 3
Various Methods for Sampling the Endometrium

Author	Total cases of Endometrial ca examined	Reported Accuracy (%)	Method of Sampling
Gravlee (1969)	56	95	Jet washer
Hecht (1956)	52	92	Aspiration
Fox et al (1962)	12	92	Brush
Morton et al (1959)	46	87	Lavage
McGuire (1962)	38	94	Novak curette

TABLE 4
Comparative Endometrial Sampling Techniques (with D & C or Subsequent Hysterectomy)

Author	Method	Accuracy Endometrial ca	Hyperplasia	No. of Patients
Ferenczy & Gelfaud (1984)	Endocyte	100%	80%	180
Grimes (Literature Review 1982)	Vabra aspiration	96%		1123
Bibbo et al (1982)	Vakutage	93%	88%	
	Endocervical aspiration	68%	14%	840
	(VCE) smears	67%	14%	
Sugimoto (1975)	Hysteroscopy	100%		1824
Raju & Taylor (1986)	Hysteroscopy	100%	100%	70

24

TABLE 5
Presenting Symptoms of 105 Patients who had
Inpatient Hysteroscopy

Symptoms	Number of Patients
Postmenopausal bleeding	60
Perimenopausal bleeding	22
Persistent menorrhagia	22
Vaginal discharge and postcoital bleeding	1
Total	105

TABLE 6
Analysis of Histological Findings in 105 Inpatients

	Histology	Hysteroscopy
Benign	39*	67
Hyperplasia	18	18
Malignant	20	20

*No histology in 28 patients with atrophic changes in endometrium

Screening

Screening for endometrial carcinoma has been rather disappointing. Table 3 shows some of the methods of sampling endometrium evaluated. None of these studies compared the results with a standard acceptable technique to evaluate their sensitivity. Later reports of studies to evaluate screening techniques for endometrial carcinoma, Table 4, compared the results with either a subsequent D & C or hysterectomy. The problem associated with more general use of endometrial aspiration cytology lies in the ability of cytologists to interpret the microscopic appearances. Endometrial cytology has always been regarded as difficult to interpret and its potential practical value has been questioned.

We have attempted to evaluate the value of routine hysteroscopy at St Thomas' Hospital, London using both a Storz microhysteroscope and a flexible cholydocoscope (Olympus) with CO_2 as the medium of insufflation. There were no cases of uterine perforation or subsequent pelvic infection or other complications noted. The histological findings of biopsies taken at hysteroscopy and hysteroscopic findings and a subsequent D & C or hysterectomy specimen were compared in 105 patients who were admitted to hospital for investigation of abnormal vaginal bleeding. Tables 5 and 6

TABLE 7

Presenting Symptoms of 84 Patients who had Outpatient Hysteroscopy

Symptoms	Number of Patients
Postmenopausal bleeding	24
Menorrhagia	20
Intermenstrual bleeding	12
Patient on HRT (asymptomatic)	28
Total	84

TABLE 8

Outpatient Hysteroscopy	
Number entered	84
Under GA	40
Without GA	44
Patient acceptability	P < 0.02

TABLE 9

Screening Asymptomatic Women (> 45 Years)

Author	No. of Patients	Method	No. of Patients with Endometrial Carcinoma
Koss et al (1981)	1280	Mi Mark and Isaacs cannula	8
Mencaglia et al (1984)	2900	Hysteroscopy	46

show the symptoms of these patients and the results of the histological and hysteroscopic findings respectively. The results of this study encouraged us to assess the use of hysteroscopy as a possible screening technique and an outpatient hysteroscopy was performed in 84 patients. Forty of these patients chose to have the procedure under general anaesthesia and 44 had the procedure under local anaesthesia or intravenous Medazalon. Patient acceptability and complications were analysed and the results are shown in Tables 7 and 8.

The two large studies reported screening asymptomatic women over the age of 45 years, Table 9 showed hysteroscopy picked up a large number of asymptomatic endometrial carcinomas.

The ease with which hysteroscopic examination can be performed, and its high rate of accuracy warrants its use as a routine procedure in the diagnosis, staging, assessment of tumour site and size, direct biopsying and screening of endometrial carcinoma.

REFERENCES

Bibbo M, Kluskens L, Azizi F *et al* (1982). Accuracy of three sampling technics for the diagnosis of endometrial cancer and hyperplasias. *J. Reprod. Med., 27*, 622–626.

Calkins A R, Stehman F B, Sutton G P, Reddy S, Hornback N B, Erlich C E (1986). Adenocarcinoma corpus et colli: Analysis of diagnostic variables: *Int. J. Radiat. Oncol. Biol. Phys., 12,* 911–916.

Chen S S (1985). Extra uterine spread in endometrial carcinoma clinically confined to the uterus. *Gynecol. Oncol., 21*, 23–31.

Cowles T A, Magrina J F, Masterson B J, Capen C V (1985). Comparison of clinical and surgical staging in patients with endometrial carcinoma. *Obstet. Gynaecol., 66*, 413–416.

Ferenczy A, Gelfand M M (1984). Outpatient endometrial sampling with endocyte: Comparative study of the effectiveness with endometrial biopsy. *Obstet. Gynecol., 63*, 295–302.

Fox C H, Turner F G, Johnson W L *et al* (1962). Endometrial cytology: A new technique. *Am. J. Obstet. Gynecol., 83*, 1582–1591.

Gravlee L C (1969). Jet-irrigation method for the diagnosis of endometrial adenocarcinoma. *Obstet. Gynecol., 34*, 168.

Grimes D A (1982). Diagnostic dilatation and curettage. A reappraisal. *Am. J. Obstet. Gynecol., 142*, 1–6.

Hecht E L (1956). The endometrial aspiration smear: Research status and clinical value. *Am. J. Obstet. Gynecol., 71*, 819–833.

Hofmeister F J (1974). Endometrial biopsy: another book. *Am. J. Obstet. Gynecol., 118*, 773–776.

Homesley H D, Boronow R C, Lewis J L (1977). Stage II endometrial adenocarcinoma. *Obstet. Gynecol., 49*, 604–608.

Koss L G, Schreiber K, Oberlander S G *et al* (1981). Screening of asymptomatic women for endometrial cancer. *Cancer, 57*, 681–691.

Lewis G C, Bundy B (1981). Surgery for endometrial cancer. *Cancer, 48*, 568–574.

McGuire T H (1962). Efficacy of endometrial biopsy in the diagnosis of endometrial carcinoma. *Obstet. Gynecol., 19*, 105–107.

Mencaglia L, Scarselli G, Tantini C (1984). Hysteroscopic evaluation of endometrial cancer. *J. Reprod. Med., 29*, 701–704.

Morton D G, Moore J G, Chang N (1957). Endometrial lavage as an aid in the diagnosis of carcinoma of the endometrium. *West. J. Surg. Gynecol. Obstet., 65*, 113–125.

Raju K S, Taylor R W (1986). Routine hysteroscopy for patients with a high risk of uterine malignancy. *Br. J. Obstet. Gynaecol., 93*, 1259–1261.

Silverberg E (1980). Cancer statistics. *Cancer, 30*, 23–38.

Stock R, Kanbour A (1975). Pre-hysterectomy curettage. *Obstet. Gynecol., 45*, 5: 535–541.

Sugimoto O (1975). Hysteroscopic diagnosis of endometrial carcinoma. *Am. J. Obstet. Gynecol., 121*, 105–113.

Surwit E A, Fowler W C, Rogoff E E, Jelevsek F, Parker R T, Creasman W T (1979). Stage II carcinoma of the endometrium. *Radiat. Oncol. Biol. Phys., 5*, 323–326.

Trotnow S, Becker H, Paterek E M (1978). Tumour volume of endometrial cancer and its prognostic significance. In: Endometrial Cancer. (Eds.) Brush M G, King R J B and Taylor R W. Bailliere Tindall, London, pp. 134–136.

Wallin T E, Malkasian G D, Gaffey T A, O'Brien P C, Fountain K S (1984). Stage II cancer of the endometrium: A pathologic and clinical study. *Gynecol Oncol., 18*, 1–17.

Welch W R, Scully R E (1977). Pre-cancerous lesions of the endometrium. *Hum. Pathol., 8*, 503–512.

DISCUSSION—RELATED TO DR RAJU'S PRESENTATION

Question   Can hysteroscopy also be used for staging cancer?

Raju   Yes.

Question   How can you use hysteroscopy to evaluate the depth or extent of invasion?

Raju   I do not attempt to evaluate myometrial invasion as this is not possible by hysteroscopy. Staging for Stage I and II is the most common use as these patients are usually in the early stages.

Question   Dr Raju, in your series of 70 patients where hysteroscopy was 100% reliable in diagnosing carcinoma, how many carcinomas did you detect?

Raju   Eighteen.

Question   Dr Raju, you had absolute correlation between your hyperplasias and carcinomas as diagnosed through hysteroscopy and histology. Can you differentiate between a severe atypical hyperplasia and an intra-endometrial carcinoma?

Raju   Our carcinomas were all either polypoidal or tumour tissue, clinically identifiable as carcinoma and histologically confirmed to be carcinoma.

Fox   I am astonished that you did not differentiate between the various forms of hyperplasia. Looking at an open uterus I am easily confused between a severe hyperplasia and a carcinoma, so I do not see how you can differentiate more easily using a hysteroscope than with an opened uterus directly in front of you.

Raju   Whatever we recorded clinically came back as histologically confirmed, which is the only way to evaluate a new technique.

Question   What is your experience with clear cell carcinomas?

Raju   We are looking at the receptors and biochemical changes in patients with clear cell carcinoma. In one of our prospective studies we gave all our patients with endometrial carcinoma Provera and found that of the clear cell carcinomas two had negative receptors and negative dehydrogenase enzymes following Provera treatment and these two women died quite quickly with the disease. Those patients with positive receptors and positive dehydrogenase enzymes following Provera treatment are actually alive 3 to 4 years later. Whether that makes any difference in prognosis has yet to be evaluated.

Question   Are you certain that you can get a complete scan of the entire surface of the endometrium with a hysteroscope?

Raju   Yes, unless it is acutely anteverted or retroverted, in which case the flexible hysteroscope is useful.

SURGERY OF ENDOMETRIAL CARCINOMA

J M Monaghan
Consultant Surgeon
Regional Department of Gynaecological Oncology
Queen Elizabeth II Hospital, Gateshead

Endometrial carcinoma has traditionally been treated as a relatively simple cancer. The majority of women who present with such a tumour respond to straightforward surgical management, however, the statistics for long term survival have remained unaltered for the last 20 years. There are many limitations to the identification of those patients at higher risk of metastases and to the actual identification of the metastases themselves.

Endometrial carcinoma is a tumour which presents frequently to many clinicians. The majority of patients present with tumour in its early stages, in marked contrast to such tumours as ovarian, the proportion of deaths occurring in Stage I endometrial cancer patients tends to be relatively low. This tumour mainly remains confined to the uterus (in its early stage of development) for a significant period of time. A number of studies have shown that although survival percentages are high, there are within this early stage disease, a small number of patients who die either because there is deep myometrial invasion, or poorer differentiation of the tumour.

Tumour grading is usually divided into Grades I, II and III. A well-differentiated tumour in early stage disease promises a good chance of cure. Patients at risk of metastases tend to be in the moderately differentiated, and the anaplastic or solid adenocarcinoma type.

ASSESSMENT

Ideally fractional curettage should be used to assess the actual position of the tumour within the uterus or if available hysteroscopy. It is also important to perform accurate bimanual examination at the same time in order to assess any extension from later stage disease into the parametrium or beyond. Clinical staging reveals very little about the spread characteristics of the disease as only when there is gross disease in the pelvis will it give any idea of the growth pattern.

Positive lymphangiography may be of value but false negative lymphangiography is frequently found. Ultrasound is of limited value in identifying metastatic disease and is only of any real value where there is gross nodal involvement. CT scanning has similar limitations. MRI has great possibilities. Any of these techniques in combination with fine needle aspiration can be used for a cytological assessment of metastatic disease.

Prognostic factors include the stage of the disease, age of the patient, uterine size, histology, myometrial invasion, lymph node metastases, peritoneal cytology and hormone receptors.

Creasman et al (1976) have published extensively in the last twelve years on various collaborative studies from centres in the United States and documented the spread characteristics of endometrial carinoma. They found that in early stage disease there was a significant positive peritoneal cytology rate which did not, however, appear to be related to uterine size or to the grade of the disease. There was, however, a relationship between the depth of myometrial invasion and the presence of positive peritoneal cytology. When each of these factors was related to prognosis there appeared to be no relationship between positive peritoneal cytology and an adverse prognostic factor. Many large collected series have shown that the stage of disease is related to five year survival. In disease identified at an early stage as being confined to the uterus prospects for cure are very high, with a steadily decreasing cure rate as spread occurs to the cervix and in turn to the pelvis and distant sites. Surgical staging allows a greater opportunity to accurately assess the true extent of the tumour and degree of matastatic spread and it is only then possible to accurately tailor treatment. Creasman *et al* (1976) showed that in early stage disease positive pelvic nodes are found in between 6% and 18% of patients with similar figures for the para-aortic nodes. A low metastatic rate is found with well-differentiated tumours, but this markedly increases as the tumour becomes more poorly differentiated. Similarly, when the endometrium alone is involved or there is superficial myometrial invasion a relatively low positive pelvic node rate and para-aortic node rate is found but a massive increase occurs as the myometrium is more deeply invaded (Boronow et al, 1984).

Manetta *et al* (1986) studied a series of patients, 115 with cervical carcinoma and 55 with endometrial carcinoma and looked at the presence or absence of para-aortic lymph node metastases in relationship to four year survival time. He found that the para-aortic node status was more important than the clinical stage of the disease. In early stage cervical carcinoma 86% of patients survived four years. If the para-aortic nodes were negative, Stages II, III and IV also all had high four year survivals. The differences were not significant. Similarly low survivals were found with Stage IB para-aortic node positive disease and a similar figure (again not statistically significant) was found for the later stages of disease. In endometrial carcinoma patients with early stage disease when compared with Stages II and III had near identical survivals when the para-aortic nodes were negative and similarly when the para-aortic nodes were positive. Manetta and his colleagues believed para-aortic node status to be a much better prognostic indicator than the clinical stage of the disease.

MANAGEMENT

Removal of the uterus is probably the most important factor in improving survival in endometrial carcinoma. Helen Bean in 1978 studied Stage I carcinoma of the endometrium and compared two groups of patients, one who had primary surgery plus selective post-operative irradiation and the others had traditional pre-operative intracavitary irradiation plus hysterectomy and vault irradiation. She found no real difference in survival in the two groups. In the first group where irradiation was used selectively according to degree of differentiation of the tumour and depth of myometrial invasion, approximately 70% of patients avoided the need for any radiotherapy.

There is not a great place for routine radical surgery in the management of endometrial carcinoma. There is a need to individualise and to tailor treatment accurately according to the metastatic potential of the disease. It is important pre-operatively to identify patients at high risk of nodal metastases and post-operatively to assess those patients with poor grade disease and myometrial invasion and determine whether other modalities of treatment should be added to the initial surgical management. Accurate clinical staging and accurate grading of the tumour pre-operatively is needed and ideally pre-radiotherapy in all cases. It is important that radiotherapy is not used pre-operatively because this can alter the assessment of the depth of myometrial invasion and modify the facility with which the pathologist can comment on the pattern of disease within the uterus. It is also important in those patients known to have Grade II and III disease pre-operatively that the pelvic and para-aortic nodes should be assessed in order to determine the metastatic pattern of the tumour.

Plentl and Friedman in 1971 showed that in well differentiated tumours the risk of vaginal recurrence is very small. Recurrence tends to be subcutaneous and vaginal vault cytology will frequently miss these recurrences, whereas pelvic examination will identify such tumours at a very early stage. The tumour frequently recurs in sites other than the vault, for example, in the suburethral area. Modified radical hysterectomy for patients with body carcinoma may reduce the risk of vault recurrence but is as much more extensive procedure than total abdominal hysterectomy, involving dissection of the ureters and removal of the upper third of the vagina. It has been shown that when a modified radical hysterectomy is used rather than a total abdominal hysterectomy then no major differences in vault recurrence rate are seen.

CONCLUSION

Initially I felt radical surgery had a significant place to play in the management of body carcinoma but I now incline more to the view that relatively simple central surgery with better assessment of the lymphatic metastases gives the patient a better prospect of more logical management. It is important to accurately assess the primary disease, ideally by means of fractional curettage and identify the site of the tumour and the stage of the disease. The pathology must give an indication of the grade of the tumour and for Stage I Grade I disease where the risk of pelvic and para-aortic metastases is approximately 2% to 3% there is no point in performing anything more radical than a total abdominal hysterectomy. For Stage I Grade II or III disease the level of pelvic and para-aortic lymph node metastases rises quite markedly and I would advocate total abdominal hysterectomy plus pelvic and para-aortic lymph node sampling. For Stage II disease where the tumour involves the corpus and may from time to time spread into the parametrium there may be a place for more radical primary surgery but to this should be added pelvic and para-aortic lymph node sampling. For later stage disease, Stages III and IV, central debulking of the tumour, ideally in the form of hysterectomy, plus pelvic and para-aortic node sampling, allows identification within the later stages of those patients who have disease still limited to the pelvis and are, therefore, amenable to adjuvant irradiation and those patients who have widespread disease where other methods of management can be considered.

In Stage I Grade I disease virtually all patients should be cured, good post-operative assessment of the specimen is needed and in those patients where there is deep myometrial invasion the addition of pelvic irradiation should be considered (Disaia and Creasman, 1986). Patients with positive pelvic and para-aortic nodes present difficulties in choice of treatment method. Many studies have shown that the addition of irradiation to primary surgery in patients with positive pelvic nodes in cervical carcinoma does not alter the prognosis. Unless the clinician handling these patients with carcinoma of the body of the uterus is confident to carry out an adequate pelvic and para-aortic node sampling procedure he should consider sending the patient to someone who is capable of doing just that.

REFERENCES

Bean H A, Bryant A J, Carmichael J A, Mallik A (1978). Carcinoma of the endometrium in Saskatchewan: 1966 to 1971. *Gynecol. Oncol., 6 (6),* 503–514.

Boronow R C, Morrow C P, Creasman W T, Disaia P J, Silverberg S G, Miller A, Blessing J A (1984). Surgical staging in endometrial cancer: Clinico-pathologic findings of a prospective study. *Obstet. Gynecol., 63,* 825–832.

Creasman W T, Boronow R C, Morrow C P, Disaia P J, Blessing J (1976). Adenocarcinoma of the endometrium: Its metastatic lymph node potential. *Gynecol. Oncol., 4,* 239–243.

Disaia P J, Creasman W T (1986). Management of endometrial adenocarcinoma Stage I with surgical staging followed by tailored adjuvant radiation therapy. *Clinics Obstet. Gynaecol., 13,* 751–766.

Manetta A, Delgado G, Petrilli E, Hummel S, Barnes W (1986). The significance of paraaortic node status in carcinoma of the cervix and endometrium. *Gynecol. Oncol., 23 (3),* 284–290.

Plentl A A, Friedman E A (1971). Lymphatic system of the female genitalia. The morphologic basis of oncologic diagnosis and therapy. *Major Probl. Obstet. Gynecol., 2.*

DISCUSSION–RELATED TO MR MONAGHAN'S PRESENTATION

Question Should you do para-aortic nodal biopsies on every patient coming to surgery with Stage I and Grade I disease?

Monaghan No. Creasman and Disaia's large series from centres throughout America showed very low pelvic and para-aortic node metastasis rates in Stage I and Grade I disease.

Question How would you define node sampling?

Monaghan My surgical technique involves removing a sheet of lymphatic tissue. In the pelvis I would remove all lymph nodes from the external iliac system in a sheet right the way down through the obturators into the internal iliac system. On the para-aortics I would take a sheet of nodes from just below the bifurcation of the aorta and the common iliacs, straight up past the inferior mesenterics to the renal vein.

Question Should you not then refer to it as node sampling?

Monaghan No, it is not what Ian Duncan refers to as 'berry-picking'.

Question What do negative nodes found on node sampling prove?

Monaghan My view of node sampling is not that I am trying to take out every piece of lymphatic tissue. It is not possible during lymphadenectomy to remove every piece of lymphatic tissue.

Question What is the improvement in outcome between people who do lymph node dissection and those who do not?

Monaghan We can identify a group of patients who are going to do well and cut down for that group on our use of adjuvant techniques. There has been much empirical management of body carcinoma in the past. Pre-operative radiotherapy was and is still in many places the routine, although there is no logical place for it. Many people routinely use progestogen but I do not think there is any place for that either. Many people request post-operative irradiation without any thought as to what they are irradiating. There is not much point in a patient with a solitary positive pelvic node in irradiating the pelvis if you do not know what is happening in the para-aortic region because that patient may also have positive para-aortic nodes.

Question With Stage I Grade II can you explain the rational of doing pelvic and para-aortic node sampling?

Monaghan Experimental methods of management, such as chemotherapy should be tested on patients with positive para-aortic lymph nodes who have a poor prospect of cure. Para-aortic lymph node sampling is technically not difficult with care and good training. The average gynaecologist should not do it. He should look after the 80% of the disease which is Stage I Grade I and can be identified pre-operatively and send the other 20% to those operators confident to do para-aortic lymph node sampling.

Question Mr Monaghan, does anybody nowadays close off the cervix before hysterectomy?

Monaghan There is no good evidence for closure of the cervix, packing the vagina, inserting picric acid or any other tumouricidal agent. Stanley Way put a radio-opaque material in and around the lower uterus and cervix and showed an easy route of spread through into the massive lymphatic plexus in the vagina, which explains why metastases occur anywhere in the vagina, but more frequently close to the vault and down the anterior vaginal wall. Creasman showed that positive peritoneal cytology does not alter the eventual prognosis of the patient, so clipping the tubes pre-operatively to prevent spillage from the uterus into the pelvic cavity when the uterus is squeezed is not necessary. My colleagues in Cape Town were concerned about the possibility of spillage of endometrial cancer cells at hysteroscopy. They followed up their hysteroscopies with immediate laparotomy and hysterectomy and found no relationship between positive peritoneal cytology and eventual prognosis.

Also the cuff of the vagina is part of the mythology of gynaecological surgery which is usually produced by scratching away with a swab at the most vascular part of the lateral angles of the bladder and all you tend to get is a lot of haemorrhage.

RADIOTHERAPY OF ENDOMETRIAL CARCINOMA

C A F Joslin
Professor and Head
University Department of Radiotherapy
University of Leeds

RADIOTHERAPY AS AN ALTERNATIVE TO OTHER METHODS OF TREATMENT

Much of the earlier work on the use of radiotherapy for treating endometrial cancer was done by Kottmeier (1959). He showed that patients who are technically or clinically inoperable and treated by irradiation do much worse than those fit patients who are technically and clinically operable, although the inoperable group may also include patients with more advanced disease. When technically operable patients were treated entirely by radiation the results improved although many of them were not clinically operable. When Kottmeier treated clinically operable patients with radiation the results appeared to be comparable to surgery. What Kottmeier did not do in this series was to allow for those patients who were radiation failures and who then went ahead to have radical surgical treatment. When that allowance was made the figures fell to around 63% survival at 5 years compared to 75% for surgery alone.

Similar results have been reported by others and there is very little in the way of hard data to support radiotherapy as the preferred method of primary management for endometrial cancer. However, for those patients in whom it is not possible to carry out surgery there are two primary methods of treatment available; i) uses a central line source and two vaginal ovoids as developed in Manchester and ii) is the Heyman capsule technique as developed in Stockholm. Both of these systems have been modified to provide for after loading the source into the uterus following the introduction of the appropriate source carriers, the major advantage gained being the almost total elimination of radiation exposure to staff. Of the two methods the Heymans' system (1947) is better since the uterus can be tightly packed-out with Heyman capsules and the tissues stretched. With a line source close contact between the sources and the tumour is not possible and the irradiation is not as evenly distributed as compared with the Heymans' capsule technique and tends to under-dose some parts of the uterus. Thus, for patients who are inoperable the Heymans' method offers the best chance of controlling disease. Kottmeier (1953) reported an increase in five year cure rates of 61% compared with 45% for the tandem technique.

INTRACAVITARY IRRADIATION AS AN ADJUNCT TO SURGERY, (PRE- OR POST-OPERATIVELY)

Stage I disease

Total abdominal hysterectomy is the current definitive method of managing endometrial carcinoma. The results with surgery alone against surgery combined with some form of intracavitary irradiation does not appear to be very much different. Pre-operative intracavitary irradiation will sterilise local tumour extension within the superficial myometrium but does not sterilise deeply invasive tumours. It is claimed to prevent iatrogenic metastases but delays definitive surgery and prevents accurate pathological assessment of the surgical specimen. It does not treat pelvic lymph nodes and may increase surgical complications. However, there is considerable evidence to show that it does reduce vaginal vault recurrence, Table 1.

TABLE 1
Vaginal Vault Recurrence Rates in Endometrial Cancer

Reference	Surgery Alone %	Pre-operative Intracavitary Irradiation %	Post-operative Intravaginal Irradiation %
Piver	7.5	4.5	0
Joslin	—	—	1.5
Graham	12	3	0
Rutledge	20	1.5	—

Post-operative intravaginal irradiation of the vaginal vault tissues suffers the disadvantage that tumour may have been transected and some remaining cells may become hypoxic and thereby radioresistant; post-surgical vaginal adhesions may increase due to the irradiation but is not, in my view, likely to be troublesome in any but a few patients. It does have the distinct advantage of not requiring a general anaesthetic and can be given using an intravaginal obturator after loaded with a radionuclide such as ^{137}Cs or ^{60}Co given on an outpatient basis. It also reduces vaginal vault recurrences to the same order as pre-operative irradiation, Table I.

Graham (1971) and Piver (1980) carried out randomised trials to compare surgery alone against pre-operative intracavitary irradiation or post-operative intravaginal treatment and neither showed any significant difference in survival, Table 2. They did, however, show a reduction in vaginal vault recurrence rates, which has been substantiated by many other series over the years, Table 1.

Stage II disease

Kuipers reported to the European Chemotherapy Group in 1983 that patients having pre-operative irradiation for Stage II disease appeared to do very well with a 5 year survival rate. However, a number of these patients had external beam therapy in addition to intracavitary treatment.

In conclusion, there would appear to be no difference in survival rates when either intracavitary pre-operative or intravaginal post-operative irradiation is carried out compared with surgery alone but vaginal vault recurrences are significantly reduced by radiotherapy whatever form it takes.

TABLE 2
Treatment of Endometrial Cancer

Groups	Survival	
	% 5 yrs (Piver)	%10 yrs (Graham)
Surgery	90	64
Pre-op Radium	93	76
Post-op Radium	96	81
	Not Significant	Not Significant at p = 0.05

Value of pre-operative intracavitary or post-operative intravaginal irradiation and 5 yr/10 yr survival against surgery alone as determined by controlled clinical trials.

TABLE 3
Relationship between Grading and Depth of Myometrial Invasion in Endometrial Cancer

Infiltration	No. of Cases	Grade I	Grade II & III
Superficial	65	63	2
Less than half myometrial invasion	81	69	12
More than half myometrial invasion	105	78	27
Total	251	210	41

EXTERNAL BEAM IRRADIATION AS AN ADJUNCT TO SURGERY

The majority of patients with Stage I disease have some form of myometrial invasion irrespective of differentiation (Table 3), however, the depth of invasion is related to the degree of differentiation. In about one quarter of cases the myometrial invasion is superficial and they tend to be well differentiated tumours as opposed to the deeply invasive poorly differentiated tumours which may reach the serosa. Lewis et al (1970) showed a direct relationship between tumour grade and the chance of lymph node involvement with an incidence of 5.5% for Grade I tumours as opposed to 26% for Grade III tumours. Similar results were reported by Creasman et al (1976) who also showed that the deeply invasive tumours had a nodal involvement of 43%, most of which were Grade III tumours. Thus it is possible to separate patients following histological grading or assessment of myometrial invasion into different prognostic groups.

Radiotherapy has been reported as being of value in treating the pelvic nodes either pre-operatively or post-operatively, Joslin (1985).

Pre-operative External Beam Irradiation

Salazar et al (1978) reported on a series of 155 patients with Grade II and III disease treated with external beam therapy pre-operatively and reported an 82% survival at 5 years but with surgical complications in 10% and chronic radiation problems in 5%. Gagnon et al (1979) reported a five year survival rate of 81% for Stage II disease treated with pre-operative external beam irradiation of 40–50Gy.

Post-operative External Beam Therapy

In our series (Joslin et al 1977) Stage I disease showed a statistically significant improvement compared to surgery alone when surgery is followed by external beam irradiation with a 5 year survival rate of 91%. However, a controlled clinical trial by Onsrud et al (1976) showed no significant difference in results between surgery followed by intravaginal irradiation against surgery followed by intravaginal irradiation plus external beam irradiation. Unfortunately, the results did not include a comparison against surgery alone. However, they did report that the vaginal recurrence rates were less in those patients who had external beam irradiation.

The value of external beam irradiation being effective in Grade III tumours as opposed to Grade I tumours has not been studied specifically in a controlled clinical trial. Salazar et al (1978) in a study on the effect of treatment and grading showed for Grade I lesions that the results did not improve much by the addition of either external beam or intracavitary irradiation when compared to surgery alone. However, for Grade III lesions the addition of pre-operative external beam radiotherapy followed by surgery produced a much lower pelvic failure rate compared with surgery alone.

CONCLUSION

External beam radiotherapy may well have something to offer when given either pre-operatively or post-operatively in Grade III disease, less in Grade II and has a questionable value in Grade I disease.

THE FUTURE

The priority for future clinical trials is to critically assess the value of external beam irradiation either pre-operatively on post-operatively and to stratify patients in terms of grade so that the assessment will provide answers for each sub-set of patients. Unfortunately to reach the required numbers the study would need to be at least a National study if not a European one.

REFERENCES

Creasman W T, Boronow R C, Morrow C P, DiSaia P J, Blessing J (1976). Adenocarcinoma of the endometrium: Its metastatic lymph node potential. *Gynecol. Oncol., 4*, 239–243.

Gagnon J D, Moss W T, Gabourel L S, Stevens K R (1979). External irradiation in the management of Stage II endometrial carcinoma. *Cancer*, *44*, 1247–1251.

Graham J (1971). The value of pre-operative or post-operative treatment by radium for carcinoma of the uterine body. *Surg. Gynecol. Obstet.*, *132*, 855–860.

Heyman J (1947). Improvement of results in the treatment of uterine cancer. *J. Am. Hosp. Ass.*, *135*, 412–416.

Joslin C A F (1985) Radiotherapy of the Cervix, Uterine Corpus and Ovary. In: Clinical Gynaecological Oncology Ed. Shepherd & Monaghan. Pub. Blackwell Scientific Pub. London.

Joslin C A F, Vaishampayan G V, Mallik T (1977). The treatment of early cancer of the corpus uteri. *Radiology*, *50*, 38–45.

Kottmeier H L (1953). Carcinoma of the Female Genitalia. Williams & Wilkins, Baltimore.

Kottmeier H L (1959). Carcinoma of the corpus uteri: diagnosis and therapy. *Am. J. Obstet. Gynecol.*, *87*, 1127.

Kuipers T J (1983). Private communication.

Lewis B V, Stallworthy J A, Cowdell (1970). Adenocarcinoma of the body of uterus. *J. Obstet. Gynaecol. Br. Commonw.*, *77*, 343–348.

Onsrud M, Kolstad P, Normann T (1976). Post operative external pelvic irradiation in carcinoma of the corpus Stage I: a controlled clinical trial. *Gynecol. Oncol.*, *4*, 222–231.

Piver M S (1980). Stage I endometrial carcinoma: The role of adjunctive radiation therapy. *Int. J. Radiat. Oncol. Biol. Phys.*, *6*, 367–368.

Rutledge F N, Tan S K, Fletcher G M (1958). Vaginal metastasis from adenocarcinoma of the corpus uteri. *Am. J. Obstet. Gynecol.*, *75*, 167–174.

Salazar O M, Feldstein M L, De Papp E W, Bonfiglio T A, Keller B E, Rubin P, Rudolph J H (1978). The management of clinical Stage I endometrial carcinoma. *Cancer*, *41*, 1016–1026.

DISCUSSION–RELATED TO PROFESSOR JOSLIN'S PRESENTATION

Question What percentage of patients treated with additional radiotherapy had morbidity such as dyspareunia or bladder problems?

Joslin There have been very few bladder problems with the doses of radiation we have been using. However, we have seen chronic proctitis in a number of these patients and one or two recto-vaginal fistulae, particularly in older women. By far the commonest morbidity is vaginal occlusion particularly when one uses external beam radiotherapy plus post-operative intravaginal treatment. This particularly applies to patients who do not have regular sexual intercourse and when they do attempt intercourse then have bleeding and dyspareunia. In those women having regular intercourse, the problems of dyspareunia are similar to those reported by women who have ongoing vaginal skin atrophy following a natural menopause. Of course many women are in this age group when they have their endometrial cancers and suffer the additional effects of irradiation.

Question Professor Joslin, is it correct to say that radiotherapy does not affect five year survival but reduces the incidence of vaginal recurrence?

Joslin External beam irradiation is reported by Allders in a controlled clinical trial to have no effect on 5 year survival. However, others including myself report that it does and this particularly applies to those with deep myometrial invasion, irrespective of grade because I do not have that data. However, there is a correlation between grade and depth of myometrial invasion in a large percentage of patients and one might expect Grades II and III to benefit more.

Question   Does irradiation reduce vaginal recurrence?

Joslin   There is sufficient evidence to show that all types of irradiation—external beam, pre-operative intracavitary and post-operative intravaginal irradiation reduce vaginal vault recurrence.

Question   Professor Joslin, why does one give differential doses of radiation to the vaginal and pelvic side wall in poor prognosis post-operative patients?

Joslin   Tissues should be taken to a level acceptable in terms of morbidity. The pelvic side wall can only be taken up to a certain dose with external beam therapy because of the limitation and morbidity to gut, in particular small gut. The vaginal vault tissues are particularly radio-resistent and if localised therapy is used in the form of intracavitary therapy there will be a rapid fall off in dose and therefore a higher local dose compared with external beam therapy can be given.

HORMONES AND CHEMOTHERAPEUTIC AGENTS IN THE MANAGEMENT OF ENDOMETRIAL CARCINOMA

R W Taylor

Professor of Obstetrics and Gynaecology

St Thomas' Hospital Medical School, London

Chemotherapy, at present, does not have value in treating endometrial carcinoma. Endometrial carcinoma arises from what is the prime oestrogen target tissue, so one would expect some of these tumours to respond to hormone therapy. Which patients to treat requires a decision on whether treatment should be confined to late disease and recurrence and whether there is a place for hormones as adjuvant therapy.

Hormone therapy has been in use for 25 years. A response rate in the region of 30–40% is expected in treatment of recurrent metastatic disease, although as metastases are not usually biopsied the type of tumour being treated is not known. There is evidence generally that metastases in endometrial carcinoma are very similar to the primary tumour. A study resulted from an international workshop at St Thomas' in 1977 in which recurrent endometrial carcinoma was treated with medroxyprogesterone acetate. A total of 120 patients with a mean age of 60 were entered in the study. Thirty-five percent were premenopausal at the time of their primary. Only 4 out of the 120 had been exposed to oestrogen before developing the primary tumour.

All patients were treated with 100 milligrammes twice daily of medroxyprogesterone acetate, for life. For patients who developed a recurrence a number of factors gave either a good or poor prognosis. With metastases in the lungs or ribs there was a response in all cases, defined as either a total disappearance of the metastases according to the criteria used in diagnosis or shrinkage of at least one third in size of the tumour. With metastases in the pelvic bones only 25% responded and with soft tissue metastases in the pelvis and abdomen few responded. The smaller the metastases the more likely partial or total response. Among the responders five patients had a total response lasting between 4 and 5 years, equal to the length of follow-up. Two patients clinically free from tumour for 2 years or more spontaneously stopped taking MPA, developed recurrent disease and subsequently died.

Despite the length of treatment there is no guarantee that all the malignancy will have been eliminated. On reviewing the response to progesterone in the different grades of tumours, Grade I tumours do best and the less differentiated tumours do relatively badly. It may not be so accurate a statement now that the better the degree of differentiation the more hormone responsive is the tumour. There is a relationship between histological grade of the tumour and hormone response but it is not nearly as close as once thought. Oestrogen encourages cell replication. It also develops the formation of more oestrogen receptor, so that the more a cell is stimulated with oestrogen the more responsive it becomes to oestrogen; and it develops the progesterone receptor, which explains why you do not get a progesterone response until you first stimulate a cell with oestrogen.

In theory, by giving oestrogen you could increase the amount of progesterone receptor in a cell and, therefore, increase progesterone sensitivity. For practical purposes that cannot be done in tumours because it encourages the growth of the tumour. However, other compounds such as tamoxifen can be given which do not enhance the growth of the tumour but actually produce progesterone receptor. There is a possibility that you may be able to change the nature of the hormone sensitivity of some tumour cells. Progesterone tends to enhance function in the endometrial cells; it blocks or partially blocks the transfer of oestrogen into the cell nucleus and promotes cell function by stimulation of the cell nucleus itself. Free oestrogen latches on to the site of the plasmic receptor; it is transmitted into the nucleus and brings about cell replication by a whole series of biochemical steps and it produces the progesterone receptor which makes the cell then responsive to progesterone.

When this sensitive cell is stimulated with progesterone a number of enzymes develop, and two that are relatively easy to measure are isocitric dehydrogenase and oestradiol dehydrogenase. The presence of these enzymes has been demonstrated within six hours of the first dose of oral MPA and is a very useful indicator of sensitivity to progesterone. The other indices used are the presence of oestrogen and progesterone receptor but these measurements are much more complicated and open to experimental error. On comparing the receptor phenotypes of endometrial carcinoma and primary breast cancer, endometrial carcinoma is much more likely to have both oestrogen and progesterone receptors than the breast primary.

With oestrogen receptor positive tumours there is a good response to progestogens such as Provera but it is not absolute. Oestrogen negative tumours do not respond at all. Progesterone positive tumours have a much higher level of response but again it is not absolute. The measurement of enzymes such as oestradiol dehydrogenase and isocitric dehydrogenase might actually give a better idea of sensitivity to progestogens than the measurement of the receptor itself.

In conclusion, our large study of 120 patients with recurrent disease shows that the previous reports in the literature, usually on very much smaller series, were rather more optimistic than has been shown to be justifiable in our series. The dosage of progestogen used is important rather than the actual type of hormone used. There is every prospect that one can change the nature of the tumour in the sense of sensitivity to progestogen. It is vital when doing biochemical analysis to know what you are biopsying. You need to be able to biopsy a tumour repeatedly, because if on biopsy you find what appears to be an insensitive tumour and you are going to try and alter the nature of that tumour you have to be able to carry out another biopsy and be reasonably sure that you obtain a comparable sample.

DISCUSSION—RELATED TO PROFESSOR TAYLOR'S PRESENTATION

Question Professor Taylor, if you had a 35 year old lady on Provera for a radical hysterectomy five years previously who presents with acne and depression, would you consider combined hormone treatment.

Taylor Hormone replacement of a combined variety is usually indicated in young women.

41

GENERAL DISCUSSION

Question What would you do with a woman with a very late menopause who is still menstruating regularly at 56 years. Would you curette repeatedly, do a hysterectomy, or disregard it as a risk factor?

Whitehead Allow her to continue to bleed.

Symonds I see very few women who menstruate after 52 or 53 years. Unless you have evidence that carcinomas are developing you should leave well alone.

Raju I would do hysteroscopy.

Question Mr Monaghan, do you pick up vaginal recurrence on vaginal screening or clinical examination.

Monaghan A careful clinical examination is most important. Although many recurrences occur in the vault, a significant number occur in other parts of the vagina which would not normally be smeared. Recurrences mainly develop subcutaneously initially and only erode through and desquamate cells at a relatively late stage. The vagina has a very complex lymphatic plexus which explains the occurrence of metastases almost anywhere.

Joslin I should like to point out that previous external beam radiotherapy should not prevent referral to the radiotherapist for a further opinion because surgical management of the lower third of the vagina is not straightforward, particularly sub-urethral.

Monaghan Radiotherapy is important in management of recurrent disease and surgery mainly in diagnosis. Many recurrences are so localised that they can be dealt with either by specific vaginal moulds with shielding or by local implantation with radiotherapeutic agents.

Joslin Radiotherapy is an important consideration in terms of interstitial implants for localised recurrence in the lower third of the vagina and in particular the sub-urethral region.

Question What is the best treatment for operable patients with Stage I disease and very little penetration, Stage I with more than one third penetration of the myometrium and Stage II patients?

Joslin For Grade I patients with superficial disease, the most likely recurrence is in the vaginal vault and the chance of that happening in good surgical hands with a reasonable vaginal cuff is probably only about 2 or 3%. At worst it is around 10 to 12%. The only argument for post-operative irradiation in that patient is for vaginal vault irradiation and external beam therapy offers us further value. If irradiation is restricted to the upper three or four centimetres of vagina morbidity can be reduced. With more than a third depth of myometrial invasion, in particular invasion towards the serosa, I irradiate the whole pelvis irrespective of the grade and give a vaginal vault irradiation as a boost following external beam irradiation. For Grade II and III disease irrespective of superficial, minimal or deep invasion, I irradiate the whole pelvis. For Stage II disease I irradiate the whole pelvis and consider the value of proceeding to radical surgery. If the patient is unsuitable for surgery I give intra-cavitary irradiation.

Monaghan   Minor variations in response to external beam irradiation may be due to micro-metastases on the pelvic side wall. For Stage I Grade I disease I advocate total abdominal hysterectomy. Those patients with deep myometrial invasion should have pelvic irradiation. For Stage II disease I advocate radical hysterectomy plus pelvic and para-aortic lymph node sampling. The 30% or so patients with positive pelvic and para-aortic lymph nodes need totally different management. You need to consider irradiation of the pelvis plus the para-aortic lymph nodes; and acceptance of the high morbidity rates from this irradiation; or the possibility of intra-operative irradiation. This is a group of patients at very poor risk who require experimental methods of management. The remainder who are lymph node negative have a very good prospect of cure.

   Seventy-five to 80% of patients are managed by the first person that sees them, which with accurate assessment of the uterus by good fractional curettage and hysteroscopy, if available, is satisfactory for Stage I Grade I disease. If at post-operative assessment there is myometrial spread, a radiotherapist should continue management. Patients with Stage II disease should be referred to a combined clinic for a gynaecological, oncology and radiotherapy opinion.

Question   Is central pelvic recurrence curable when the patient has not had radiotherapy? Does lower vaginal recurrence denote a much worse prognosis than superficial recurrence at the vaginal vault?

Joslin   The prognosis for sub-urethral recurrence is not necessarily bad. In some cases a solitary metastasis responds extremely well to a localised interstitial implant. However, the recurrence must be small to benefit from an effective cancericidal dose. If a vaginal vault recurrence is small and superficial it may be possible to control the tumour with intravaginal irradiation. Larger lesions require external beam irradiation. If your patient is fit and suitable, it is worth giving external beam therapy to the whole pelvis.

Monaghan   If radiotherapy does not completely clear the lesion, or there is persistent recurrence at the same site you should consider exenterative surgery.

Question   What is the optimal means of managing a patient with nodal disease?

Monaghan   Are we effectively dealing with Stage IV disease?

Reply   Yes

Monaghan You improve the prospects for this patient if you remove the central disease and use adjuvant therapy to the pelvic side wall. At present the best option is irradiation but whether that is pre-surgery or post-surgery is important to discuss. If the surgery is essentially a central de-bulking total abdominal hysterectomy then from the data Professor Joslin has, pre-operative external beam irradiation may be the best option.

A sophistication of pelvic and para-aortic lymph node assessment is the extra-peritoneal technique for removing nodes without invading the peritoneal cavity. Extra-peritoneal lymph node assessment can provide much more information with minimal morbidity to the patient and then allow the use, with great confidence and a low morbidity of radical radiotherapeutic techniques.

Joslin I agree, that has been the finding of our overseas colleagues, although we do not have much experience in this country of that technique. I am very cynical about the value of radiotherapy once the disease is in the para-aortic nodes, when it almost invariably indicates systemic spread of disease.

I normally restrict management to the pelvis. Even if I could reduce local recurrence in the para-aortic nodes, the patient still tends to die of their disease at other sites.

Taylor With disease where ultimately you may need to use progestogens later, you must determine whether it is a sensitive tumour. There are ways to enhance tumour sensitivity, such as the use of tamoxifen.

Joslin Does anyone in the audience routinely give adjuvant progestogens following surgery and/or radiotherapy for endometrial cancer?

Audience Yes

Joslin Why?

Audience It is probably an emotional response on my part but I give the progesterone to them all and have not found that it does any harm at all. I had one patient who stopped her progesterone and the tumour recurred and I never got on top of it again.

Monaghan The Leeds and Oslo studies showed that the actual deaths in the group treated with progestogens and the untreated group were identical. It is time for real studies on the use or non-use of progestogens.

LIST OF DELEGATES

B R Y Abeywardena
Hemel Hempstead

Z O Amarin
London

H Awad
Bolton

G A Ayida
London

O M Aziz
London

S C Bamber
Newmarket

V L Barley
Bristol

D M Barrett
Pembury

T Beedham
London

H Bharucha
Belfast

A Bigrigg
Bristol

J T Blair
Glasgow

K E Blake
Lewes

W A H Bodger
Canterbury

T H Bourne
Gloucester

P M Bousquet
London

J Browning
Oxford

H M B Busfield
Derby

M P Cahir
London

P J Callen
Truro

P A Canney
Birmingham

H Cole
Northampton

C Coulter
London

J W Crawford
Dundee

R Crawford
London

J Crow
London

A E Davies
Cranbrook

J A K Davies
Dyfed

A Driscoll
Guildford

L Duley
Oxford

M Edwards
Basingstoke

K H Eltom
Lincoln

J Fairbank
London

N J Faruqi
Barking

D J C Felton
Cambridge

M A Flaherty
London

M L Forman
Manchester

O A Ghani
Shrewsbury

C A Gie
Nottingham

K A Godfrey
Sunderland

B W Hackman
Peterborough

R H Hammond
Oxbridge

R Jelley
London

D Jesinger
Southampton

L I Khaleel
Truro

S Khanna
Leicester

A I Kiwanuka
Salford

R W Laing
London

H E Lambert
London

D A S Lawrence
Luton

A Lesseps
Poole

45

D T Y Liu
Nottingham

M Longin
Gravesend

I Z Mackenzie
Oxford

I W Manson
Preston

A McCartan
London

J McCormack
Birmingham

J McGarry
Barnstable

F S B Melkonian
Barnsley

O Moollan
Chertsey

H Morgan
London

K A Muhombe
London

J M Mukoyogo
Birmingham

M J Muldoon
Grimsby

M N Nasri
Prescot

B C Obi
Slough

M E A O'Connel
London

C Overton
Manchester

C R Porteous
Ormskirk

J Pryse-Davies
London

D A Russell Lees
Inverness

A Samuel
Shrewsbury

U Sarma
Croydon

K S Sarvananthar
Southampton

M W Seif
Manchester

H Sharma
Hounslow

D C Shove
Barnet

S K Shrivastava
Leeds

M M Singh
Newcastle

A M Smith
Wolverhampton

G M Smith
Leicester

M R Smith
Burton on Trent

P Stone
Bristol

R P Symonds
Glasgow

C Tai
London

Y Tayob
London

V Tebbs
Southampton

J Thampi
Co. Antrim

H Thomson
Pinner

C Thornton
Belfast

N Trickey
Sunninghill

R Varma
Guildford

J Vernon-Parry
Worksop

D M Viveash
Crawley

P F Wale
Derby

A T Watson
Lincoln

A W Wheater
Manchester

D Whillis
Sheffield

A S Wilkinson
Crawley

C D A Wolfe
London

S Wonnacott
Southampton

J T Wright
Chertsey

R N Yadav
Rush Green